Praise for

CHRISTIANE NORTHRUP, M.D.

and

Women's Bodies, Women's Wisdom

"Feminine wisdom is the intelligence at the heart of creation. It is holistic, intuitive, contextual, and functions as a field of infinite correlation. Dr. Northrup's book is an expression of this wisdom."
—Deepak Chopra, M.D., author of *Ageless Body, Timeless Mind*

"*Women's Bodies, Women's Wisdom* is a gateway to the deepest understanding of health and well-being. Women have an innate sense of spirituality, an ability to attune to the wisdom within themselves and the larger whole that has been systematically ignored in medicine. Dr. Northrup restores the spiritual to the medical, facilitating the understanding and confidence that every woman needs in order to create a healthy body and a fulfilled life."
—Joan Borysenko, Ph.D., author of *Minding the Body, Mending the Mind* and *A Woman's Book of Life*

"A masterpiece for every woman who has an interest in her body, her mind, and her soul."
—Caroline Myss, Ph.D., author of *Anatomy of the Spirit*

"While most male physicians seem hesitant even to use the word 'healing,' many women doctors—epitomized by Dr. Christiane Northrup—are demonstrating what genuine healing has always been about: the integration of the physical and the spiritual, psyche and soma, into a harmonious whole. This book demonstrates the reemergence of the feminine in healing, a force that has kept the inner pulse of healing beating for centuries. If you can't have Dr. Northrup for your doctor, read her book."
—Larry Dossey, M.D., author of *Healing Words, Meaning & Medicine,* and *Recovering the Soul*

"Dr. Chris Northrup's book is an outstanding collection of information and case histories that will benefit everyone who reads it. It lives up to the title and I certainly intend to share it with my wife and daughter. I could go on extolling its virtues, but it will do more good if everyone just takes my advice and reads it."
—Bernie Siegel, M.D., author of *Love, Medicine, and Miracles*

The Wisdom of Menopause is a
Featured Alternate Selection of
Book-of-the-Month Club and an
Alternate Selection of One Spirit Book Club